MELT METHOD FOR PAIN RELIEF

A Complete Guide For Unlocking The Body's Healing Wisdom And Effective Approach To Pain Management

WALTER ZYAIRE

No part of this book may be reproduced, stored in a retrieval system, or transmitted in any form or by any means, electronic, mechanical, photocopying, recording, or otherwise, without the express written permission of the author, with the exception of small extracts in critical reviews or articles.

DISCLAIMER

The information in this book is intended only for general informational purposes; it should not be used in lieu of professional advice or medical care. Since the author is not licensed to practice therapy, the information offered should not be used in place of the expertise, judgment, or guidance of qualified mental health or medical professionals. Readers are encouraged to consult therapists, medical specialists, or other qualified authorities regarding their particular situation and needs. The publisher and author disclaim all liability for any actions or decisions taken by readers based on the information in this book. Results may vary from person to person and this book's approaches, procedures, and strategies may not be suitable in all circumstances. Considering unique situations and consulting a qualified expert are essential when choosing the right course of action. Neither the publisher nor the author recommend or guarantee the efficacy of any therapy or treatment that is indicated in this book. Because the information is based on the author's research and understanding at the time of publishing, it could not reflect the most recent developments or practices in the treatment area. The publisher and the author both disclaim all liability for the accuracy, completeness, or use of the material in this book. Readers bear full responsibility for the decisions and actions they choose in light of the information presented in this book.

TABLE OF CONTENTS

ABOUT THE BOOK

The pioneering book The MELT Method for Pain Relief explores the science and practical applications of the MELT technique, providing readers with a thorough grasp of how this approach can change their lives. The book introduces readers to the MELT environment and lays the groundwork for a discussion of pain and the significant effects of the MELT approach. The book's format, which includes an examination of the neurofascin system and the intriguing relationship between connective tissue and pain, is thoughtfully crafted to lead readers through the science underlying MELT.

For readers who are just starting their MELT journey, it offers crucial information on setting up a secure practice area, preparing, and tools. The book covers the fundamental MELT techniques, which lay the groundwork for the next chapters on MELT applications for other body areas.

These techniques include the Roller Foot Treatment, Soft Ball Hand Treatment, and Basic Neck Release.

With a focused approach, it covers pain management methods for several body parts, including the back, hips, knees, neck, and shoulders. Readers are then given instructions on how to use MELT in daily activities, including using it for stress relief and relaxation as well as incorporating it into workout regimens.

The holistic side of MELT is examined, which also covers how it affects energy levels, intestinal health, and the quality of sleep. The book highlights the integration of mindfulness and MELT, emphasizing the use of MELT as a meditation tool, attentive breathing, and the mind-body connection.

For those looking for a revolutionary approach to pain management and general well-being, The MELT Method for Pain Relief offers an organized and thorough manual.

CHAPTER ONE

OVERVIEW OF THE MELT METHOD FOR PAIN RELIEF

GREETINGS FROM THE MELT WORLD!

Take a trip through time as we explore the world of MELT, a cutting-edge approach to holistic well-being that transcends traditional health and fitness practices. Myofascial Energetic Length Technique, or MELT for short, is a novel and distinct method for treating pain and enhancing bodily function. This approach highlights the complex relationship between the myofascial system and general physical well-being and provides a complete solution for improved vitality and long-lasting relief.

KNOWLEDGE OF PAIN AND THE MELT APPROACH

A thorough grasp of pain and its intricate link to the myofascial system is fundamental to the MELT philosophy. Targeting the connective tissues that pervade the body, MELT goes beyond existing methods that frequently concentrate only on symptom treatment to address the underlying causes of pain. The myofascial system, which is made up of muscles and fascia, is essential to preserving body integrity and sustaining physiological processes. The MELT Method seeks to alleviate pain and enhance overall well-being by releasing tension, restoring balance, and improving alignment in the myofascial system through a series of specific methods and exercises.

MELT encourages people to take an active role in their recovery by emphasizing the need for self-care. MELT promotes an intentional approach to well-being that goes beyond the time spent performing a particular exercise or session by raising awareness of the body's natural capacity for healing and regeneration. With guidance, participants examine their bodies, paying attention to the tiny signs that may indicate regions of imbalance or tension. A key component of the MELT

Method is this increased self-awareness, which promotes a stronger bond between the mind and body.

HOW YOUR LIFE CAN BE CHANGED BY MELT

The potential for transformation that comes with MELT goes well beyond only relieving physical pain; it also includes improving one's whole quality of life comprehensively.

Through treating the root causes as well as the symptoms, MELT's multimodal approach promotes long-lasting gains in mental, emotional, and physical health. People who start the MELT journey may experience a renewed sense of energy, resilience to everyday stressors, and a renewed sense of vitality.

In addition, MELT is made to be usable by people of various ages and fitness levels. MELT provides a flexible and adaptable solution for anyone trying to improve performance as an athlete, manage chronic pain, or just take a proactive approach to well-being.

People can develop a robust and well-balanced body via consistent practice, which opens up possibilities for a more lively and satisfying existence.

Discover the profound ways that MELT may positively impact and revolutionize your life as we delve into the nuances of pain and the myofascial system. Discover the transformational potential of MELT.

CHAPTER TWO

THE MELT SCIENCE

THE INTRIGUING LINK BETWEEN PAIN AND CONNECTIVE TISSUE

The fascinating link between connective tissue and pain is one of the basic ideas investigated in the science of MELT. The intricate web of fibers known as connective tissue gives different organs and tissues structural support. It is essential to preserving the integrity of the body. Its role in pain perception is becoming more and more evident in research.

MELT emphasizes the importance of treating this sometimes disregarded component of the body's structure by arguing that connective tissue disorder may be a factor in pain and discomfort. Beyond traditional approaches, MELT offers a comprehensive approach to pain management by recognizing and addressing the connection between pain and connective tissue health.

EXAMINING THE NERVOUS SYSTEM

The investigation of the neurofascial system is a fundamental component of MELT science. The complex interaction between the neurological system and the fascial network—the connective tissue that encases and supports muscles and organs—is referred to as the neurofascial system. MELT acknowledges the role this system plays in controlling mobility, range of motion, and general health. MELT looks at the neurofascin system to find and treat underlying problems that might be causing pain and limited movement. This thorough method offers a sophisticated view of the body's functional anatomy by acknowledging the dynamic link between neurological impulses and fascial integrity.

WHY MELT IS EFFECTIVE: THE METHOD'S SCIENTIFIC BASIS

Deciphering the scientific tenets that underlie MELT is necessary to comprehend why the approach is effective. The reason that MELT works so well is because it can affect the autonomic nervous system and encourage a change from the tense, stress-inducing sympathetic state to the relaxed, parasympathetic state. This change has a significant impact on the body's capacity to mend and rebalance. MELT aims to improve tissue quality generally by promoting hydration and targeting the connective tissue with mild, specialized treatments. The approach encourages people to take an active role in their well-being by emphasizing self-care and self-treatment. Furthermore, MELT recognizes the brain's ability to change and reorganize in response to sensory input by incorporating the principles of neuroplasticity. This neuroscientific basis emphasizes how regular practice of MELT can lead to beneficial, long-lasting improvements. MELT essentially uses a thorough understanding of connective tissue, neurofascial dynamics, and neurological response to support general well-being, in line with the body's natural ability to heal itself.

CHAPTER THREE

BEGINNING TO USE MELT

GETTING READY FOR YOUR MELT ADVENTURE

It takes careful planning before starting your MELT journey to guarantee a successful and enjoyable experience. Myofascial Energetic Length Technique, or MELT for short, is a self-care technique that targets the connective tissue system to enhance flexibility, balance, and general well-being. It's crucial to comprehend the fundamental ideas of MELT and its possible advantages before you begin.

Start by being acquainted with the fundamental ideas of MELT. Using tiny balls and specialized soft foam rollers, the method applies light pressure to various body parts to encourage the release of fascial tissue and hydration. Your appreciation of MELT and its possible effects on your body will grow if you comprehend how the technique functions physiologically.

Take into account your health and any underlying medical issues. Before beginning MELT, it is advisable to speak with a healthcare provider about any worries or medical conditions you may have. Although most people find MELT to be gentle, customized guidance guarantees that you can customize the technique to your unique requirements and constraints.

CRUCIAL INSTRUMENTS AND HARDWARE

Purchasing the appropriate instruments and apparatus is essential to the success of a MELT practice. Little balls and soft foam rollers are the main instruments used in MELT, and each has a specific function. Soft foam rollers are available in various densities; it's important to select the one that will be most comfortable for you. When they are just starting, beginners might choose a gentler roller and work their way up to firmer ones.

To target smaller areas and joints, it is also imperative to get a set of MELT Method balls.

These balls apply exact pressure to relieve tension in targeted places, imitating the hands-on techniques used in MELT. To fit various body parts, including hands, feet, and the neck, it is advised to have a range of ball sizes.

ESTABLISHING A SECURE AND COSY ENVIRONMENT FOR MELT

To get the most out of your MELT practice, you must set up a comfortable and devoted area. Select a place that is calm, well-lit, and free of distractions so that you can concentrate on the exercises. Make sure there are no possible hazards in the area so that your practice can be conducted in a safe atmosphere.

When performing workouts, place the foam roller on a non-slip mat or carpet to keep it stationary. This improves stability and guarantees that you can confidently execute MELT exercises. To improve the entire experience of your MELT session, think about utilizing essential oils or playing relaxing music to create a tranquil ambiance.

 Be mindful of the clothes you wear. Put on loose, airy clothing that doesn't restrict your freedom of motion. This guarantees unrestricted execution of MELT exercises, fostering a more pleasurable and productive practice.

 You may create an environment that is conducive to a transforming and gratifying experience by setting up a conducive place, investing in the necessary tools, and emotionally and physically preparing for your MELT trip. MELT can improve your entire health, and making careful preparations will guarantee that you can get the full benefits of this treatment.

CHAPTER FOUR

THE FUNDAMENTAL MELT METHODS

THE HAND TREATMENT WITH A SOFT BALL

One essential part of the MELT approach is the Soft Ball Hand Treatment, which targets wrist and hand tension and discomfort. This method encourages the release of stored-up tension and enhances general hand function by using a softball to gently push on particular hand locations. The Soft Ball Hand Treatment attempts to relieve the pain associated with arthritis, repetitive strain, and other hand-related conditions by focusing on important areas, including the palm, fingers, and wrists. Enhancing overall well-being and hand movement fluidity are the goals of this practice.

THE FOOT ROLLER THERAPY

The Roller Foot Treatment, which targets tension and tightness in the feet and lower limbs, is another essential component of the MELT treatment.

This method, which targets different pressure points, entails rolling the foot over the surface of a soft foam roller. When someone has plantar fasciitis or general foot weariness, the Roller Foot Treatment can be especially helpful as it helps release accumulated stress and discomfort in the feet. Improved posture and general body alignment are benefits of this treatment, which increases the flexibility and mobility of the foot.

THE FUNDAMENTAL RELEASE OF THE NECK

One of the fundamental MELT techniques, the Basic Neck Release, focuses on relieving tension in the shoulders and neck. The Basic Neck Release seeks to reduce stiffness and pain in the neck region by using mild compression and elongation techniques. This method is particularly helpful for people who have stiffness from bad posture, tension headaches, or neck pain. The Basic Neck Release helps to create a better general alignment, lessen the chance of persistent neck problems, and promote relaxation and increased range of motion in the neck.

OVERVIEW OF MELT FOOT AND HAND TREATMENTS

The Hand and Foot Treatments, a crucial part of MELT, offer a thorough method for enhancing general well-being. These treatments offer a special blend of self-massage and mild compression techniques, going beyond conventional self-care practices. The connective tissue abnormalities that can cause pain and discomfort in the hand and foot regions are the focus of the MELT Hand and Foot Treatments. People who incorporate these treatments into their self-care routines can report improvements in their mobility, decreased discomfort, and increased awareness of their bodies. A comprehensive approach to self-care that promotes general health and well-being is built upon the MELT Hand and Foot Treatments.

CHAPTER FIVE

MELT FOR VARIOUS BODY AREAS

SHOULDERS AND NECK: RELAXING TENSION

The MELT technique addresses the often-ignored connective tissue, or fascia, to offer a comprehensive method of releasing tension in the neck and shoulders. MELT seeks to hydrate the fascial system, promoting greater flexibility and reducing stiffness, using several gentle yet effective treatments.

People can target particular neck and shoulder regions with soft body rollers and specialty balls, which help to relieve tension and encourage relaxation. In addition to highlighting the value of self-care, MELT gives people the tools they need to actively manage their health and offers a workable and approachable way for people to relieve stress in these frequently impacted areas.

BACK PAIN: A WHOLESOME METHOD

MELT is a holistic approach to treating back pain, emphasizing the spine's mobility and stability. To improve the body's inherent healing processes, the technique places a strong emphasis on rehydrating connective tissue. People can reduce muscular imbalances, enhance their posture, and ease lower back stress by combining several MELT treatments. To strengthen the core muscles and give the spine long-term stability, the MELT approach also includes targeted movements and exercises. For those looking for alleviation and increased functionality, MELT provides a comprehensive and efficient approach by addressing both the structural and neuromuscular aspects of back pain.

KNEE AND HIP PAIN: REGAINING MOVEMENT

Recognizing the body's interdependence, MELT uses targeted strategies to restore mobility to treat hip and knee discomfort.

MELT facilitates the release of tension, enhancement of range of motion, and mitigation of discomfort by focusing on the fascial network encircling the hips and knees. People can apply light pressure to important regions, improving alignment and lessening joint stress, by using MELT balls and soft body rollers. The technique also includes strengthening exercises to improve muscular support, offering a comprehensive strategy for regaining hip and knee mobility and function.

FOOT AND ANKLE PROBLEMS: GETTING HELP

MELT provides focused pain and discomfort relief for people with foot and ankle problems. MELT seeks to improve general foot health, decrease inflammation, and increase flexibility by targeting the connective tissue in the feet and ankles. The treatment stimulates the release of stress and enhances circulation by targeting the soles of the feet with particular MELT ball techniques. In addition, MELT offers exercises to strengthen the muscles that support the feet and stresses the significance of appropriate foot alignment, providing a comprehensive approach to alleviating common foot and ankle issues.

HAND AND WRIST PAIN: MELT REMEDIES

By focusing on the fascial network and encouraging improved hand and wrist health, MELT offers practical treatments for reducing discomfort in the hands and wrists. People can relieve wrist and hand tension and symptom relief, including pain and stiffness, by using MELT hand and foot treatments. The technique also includes targeted workouts to strengthen grip and increase wrist joint stability. Through the treatment of soft tissues and joint function, MELT provides a useful and approachable method for relieving hand and wrist pain, enabling people to actively participate in their health and well-being.

CHAPTER SIX

INCLUDING MELT IN YOUR EVERYDAY ACTIVITIES

CREATING YOUR CUSTOMIZED MELT SCHEDULE

Personalized MELT (Myofascial Energetic Length Technique) routines are made by assessing your body's demands and modifying the exercise to target trouble spots. First, determine which major areas—such as stiff neck, lower back pain, or tight shoulders—may benefit from MELT. After you've identified these areas, create a plan that addresses each one in turn.

To prime your body for the upcoming procedures, start your MELT program with a mild warm-up. This could involve deep breathing techniques or gentle stretches to encourage relaxation. Use the basic MELT procedures, such as the Hand and Foot Treatments, to start releasing tension in the body's connective tissue, as well.

To keep track of your development and pinpoint areas that need more work, think about including self-assessment tools like the MELT Map. Continually review and adjust your regimen in light of your changing needs. Your MELT routine's ability to prevent chronic tension and promote general well-being will be enhanced if you can make it more consistent.

INCLUDING MELT IN YOUR WORKOUT ROUTINE

To maximize the advantages of your current workout regimen and reduce the risk of injury, MELT can be easily included. Use MELT as a pre-workout program to get your body ready for movement before moving on to more strenuous exercise. Merely applying MELT can maximize your range of motion and enhance muscle efficiency when you work out by correcting fascial imbalances and releasing tension.

To keep your muscles supple and avoid muscle fatigue, think about using MELT techniques in between sets or exercises during your workout. Activities that require repetitive motions or high-impact stress on joints may benefit the most from this. Your performance may increase, your risk of overuse injuries may decrease, and your muscles may feel less sore after working out with MELT.

Use MELT as a post-workout recovery tool when you're done working out. This can facilitate improved circulation, ease tense muscles, and hasten the healing process. Through regular integration of MELT with your workout regimen, you can develop a comprehensive fitness regimen that targets your body's structural and energetic components.

MELT FOR RELAXATION AND STRESS REDUCTION

Apart from its health advantages, MELT is an effective method for relaxation and stress alleviation. A contemplative experience is produced by the soft, rhythmic motions of MELT, which encourage serenity and awareness. Including MELT in your daily routine can be particularly beneficial for stress management and mental health promotion.

 Throughout the day, you can utilize the Hand and Foot Treatments in particular as fast methods to relieve stress. These easy exercises relieve tension in the hands and feet, which are frequently the sites of stress expression. You can also use the MELT Soft Roller for full-body relaxation, which will help you relax and let go of tension in different muscle groups.

 To improve the quality of your sleep, think about including MELT in your evening routine. An enjoyable night's sleep can be encouraged by the relaxing effects of MELT, which can help quiet the body and mind. MELT can help you develop a comprehensive approach to well-being that takes into account both the physical and emotional elements of health when incorporated into your stress reduction techniques.

CHAPTER SEVEN

MELT FOR PARTICULAR SITUATIONS

MELT FOR THE TREATMENT OF CHRONIC PAIN

The Myofascial Energetic Length Technique, or MELT, has shown promise in the treatment of chronic pain. Chronic pain can be crippling and difficult to treat. It is typically defined as continuous discomfort that lasts longer than the anticipated time for healing. By emphasizing the myofascial system—the intricate web of muscles and fascia that is essential to preserving body function—MELT provides a distinct viewpoint.

MELT is a specialized technique that uses small balls and soft foam rollers to release tension, hydrate connective tissue, and bring the body back into equilibrium. MELT is different from traditional pain management techniques in that it places a strong emphasis on the myofascial system, giving people a comprehensive way to reduce chronic pain. Frequent application of MELT has demonstrated encouraging outcomes in terms of pain reduction and general well-being for those with ailments including fibromyalgia, arthritis, or lower back pain.

USING MELT TO ADDRESS POSTURAL ISSUES

In today's sedentary lifestyle, postural problems are common and can cause pain, discomfort, and restricted mobility. MELT targets the underlying myofascial linkages that are in charge of maintaining posture, offering a novel approach to treating postural abnormalities. By releasing tension in specific regions, the mild techniques used in MELT promote improved alignment and lessen the load on the musculoskeletal system.

Through the integration of MELT into a daily regimen, people can actively strive to enhance their posture and avoid associated problems. By encouraging a sense of awareness and connection with their body, MELT's self-care component gives people the power to take control of their health.

This method promotes long-term musculoskeletal health by acting as a preventive measure in addition to relieving current posture issues.

MELT FOR ATHLETES: IMPROVING RECUPERATION AND PERFORMANCE

Athletes are always looking for methods to improve their time to recover and maximize performance. The athletic community has come to recognize MELT as a useful technique for improving performance and hastening recuperation. The myofascial techniques used in MELT can help with joint mobility, muscle tightness reduction, and flexibility enhancement—all essential components of successful sports performance.

When it comes to healing, MELT provides a non-invasive way to treat muscular discomfort and encourage quicker healing. When athletes use MELT in their training, they can expect faster recovery times, a lower chance of injury, and increased performance all around. MELT techniques are accessible to athletes of all skill levels and can be used either alone or under the supervision of a MELT instructor, which contributes to their attractiveness as a useful and efficient tool.

MELT AND PREGNANCY: A SECURE METHOD FOR PAIN MANAGEMENT

Expectant moms experience a variety of bodily changes and discomforts during pregnancy. MELT is a safe and compassionate method of treating pain during pregnancy, taking into account the particular difficulties that come during this life-changing time. Pregnant women can improve overall well-being, reduce swelling, and ease tension without overstressing their bodies by using soft foam rollers and balls.

Because MELT focuses on the myofascial system, it can be very helpful in treating typical pregnancy-related problems like swollen feet, back pain, and pelvic discomfort. People may feel more in control of their physical well-being, sleep better, and feel more comfortable when they incorporate MELT into their pregnant self-care regimen. Before starting a MELT program, as with any wellness practice during pregnancy, it is best to speak with medical professionals to be sure it is appropriate for your specific situation.

MELT FOR WELLNESS: BEYOND PAIN RELIEF USING MELT TO IMPROVE SLEEP QUALITY

Within the field of holistic wellness, the Myofascial Energetic Length Technique (MELT) is a potentially effective means of improving the quality of sleep. This novel method addresses the myofascial system by combining soft body therapies and gentle motions to release tension and stress that could be causing sleep difficulties. The relationship between myofascial health and sleep is important because tensions in the fascial tissues can impair one's capacity to obtain restorative sleep by causing discomfort and restlessness. By utilizing its distinct approach, MELT aims to alleviate this stress, encouraging calmness and opening the door for better sleep cycles.

In addition to the physical components, mindfulness and relaxation techniques are emphasized in MELT. These are important elements in creating an environment that is favorable to getting good sleep. MELT can help people sleep better at night by promoting deeper, more restorative sleep, which is good for their general health.

INCREASING VITALITY AND ENERGY

MELT has an impact on more than just pain management; it also encompasses a comprehensive strategy to increase vigor and energy. A disruption to the myofascial system might lead to a decrease in energy levels because it is essential for maintaining total body function. By using specific MELT procedures, practitioners want to address potential energy-draining habits and bring the myofascial system back into balance.

Exercises that both relieve tension and activate the nervous system are incorporated into the practice to encourage a heightened sense of vitality. MELT improves general well-being by encouraging improved alignment and fluidity in movement, which may increase stamina and endurance. MELT is positioned as a useful tool for those looking for natural and sustainable ways to energize their bodies because of its comprehensive approach to energy management.

MELT TO IMPROVE GASTROINTESTINAL HEALTH

A key component of MELT for well-being is the complex interaction between the myofascial system and digestive function. Fascial tensions can affect how the digestive organs work, which may result in discomfort and inadequate digestion.

Using specific techniques, MELT aims to release tension and improve the organs' natural movement by targeting the myofascial connections associated with the digestive system.

Moreover, MELT emphasizes the importance of drinking for digestive health. Sufficient hydration maintains the fascial tissues' flexibility, avoiding stiffness that could obstruct digestive functions. MELT is a promising treatment for people looking to address digestive difficulties holistically because of its mild yet targeted approach. Through the promotion of a balanced and harmonious myofascial system, MELT offers a comprehensive approach to general well-being and enhances digestive health.

CHAPTER EIGHT

MINDFULNESS AND MELT

THE LINK BETWEEN MIND AND BODY IN MELT

Sue Hitzmann's MELT technique highlights the complex interrelationship between the mind and body. Fundamentally, MELT works with the body's fascia, or connective tissues, to improve this relationship. The body depends heavily on these tissues for support and stability, and the MELT approach uses specialized technology and gentle techniques to release tension in the fascial system. By doing this, MELT recognizes the significant influence that the mind may have on the body's general health in addition to promoting physical well-being.

People are encouraged to explore their body sensations mindfully through a variety of MELT exercises. By fostering a closer connection between the mind and body, this increased awareness enables people to pinpoint their points of tension or discomfort.

Thus, the MELT approach becomes a comprehensive exercise that fosters a deeper awareness of one's body by encouraging a conscious presence at the moment in addition to relieving physical discomfort.

MELT AND MINDFUL BREATHING

A key component of MELT is mindful breathing, which combines the ideas of breath awareness with the intentional release of tension in the connective tissues of the body. To improve the mind-body connection, MELT practitioners are instructed to focus on their breath and pay special attention to it. People can enhance the effects of MELT by coordinating their breathing with particular motions and exercises, which produces a synergistic impact that encourages stress reduction and relaxation.

In MELT, mindful breathing emphasizes the value of deep, diaphragmatic breaths by involving intentional inhalation and exhalation. By facilitating the release of tension within the fascial system, this deliberate breathing pattern enhances general well-being. MELT practitioners develop a mindful presence that transcends the practice, encouraging a sense of peace and awareness in daily life, as they grow attentive to their breath throughout sessions.

Using MELT as a Meditation Tool: MELT is more than just a way to work out physically; it also has applications in meditation. Including MELT in a meditation routine provides an alternative method for developing calmness and awareness. MELT exercises help people enter a meditative state by providing a concrete point of attention through deliberate and focused movements.

By encouraging practitioners to approach each action with awareness and intention, the MELT method turns yoga into a kind of moving meditation. People may center themselves while they do the purposeful and rhythmic sequences, which strengthens the bond between the body and the mind. With its focus on the fascial system, MELT's tactile nature provides a concrete foundation for meditation, offering a fresh approach to investigating the present moment and fostering mental health.

A holistic approach to well-being is facilitated by mindful breathing, the Mind-Body Connection in MELT, and using MELT as a meditation tool. Using deliberate motions, attentive breathing, and an emphasis on the fascial system, MELT transforms from a physical workout into a contemplative routine that fosters the relationship between the mind and body.